A Quick And Easy Guide To Baby Showers!

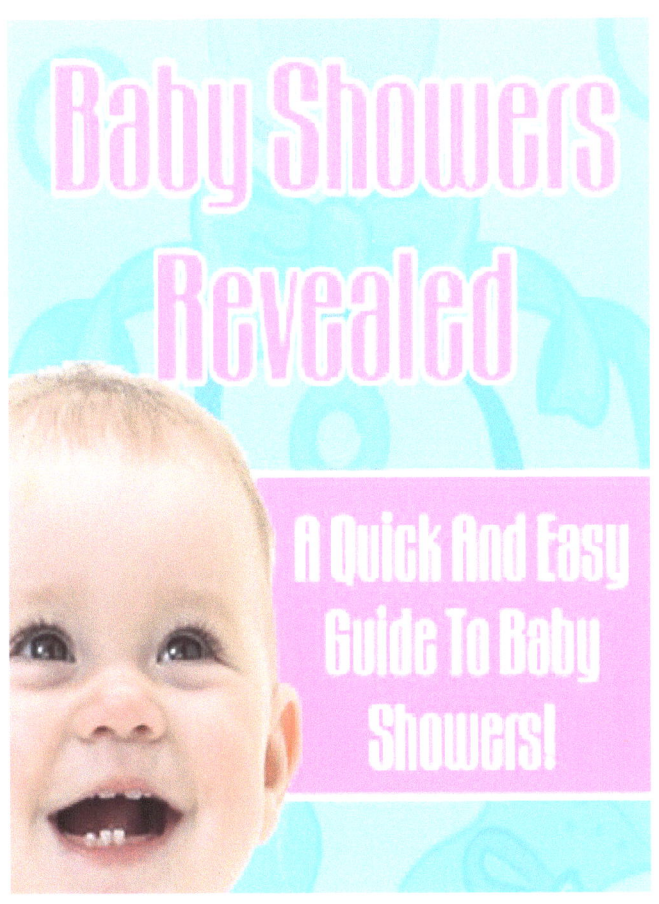

Table of Contents

INTRODUCTION

How wonderful! One of your best friends in the whole wide world has just announced that she's pregnant. Naturally, you're delighted, and can't hold back your tears of joy. It's hard to imagine that, in just a matter of time, your special friend is going to be a mother (maybe even for the second or third time...or more!).

As you let the amazing news sink in, your friend is envisioning the journey that will usher in a new life into the world: the gynecologist visits, the morning sickness, the ultrasound testing, the roller coaster of emotions that will eventually culminate in an experience that defies description.

Indeed, despite the frequency of births – tens of thousands a day, all across the world – they remain nothing short of miraculous. It's not hard to imagine, therefore, that your friend is reflecting on issues that are truly hard to put into words.

Your world, however, is rather more pragmatic. You're thinking of the baby shower; or rather, you're thinking that you might not know *enough* about planning and managing a baby shower. And that has you worried.

Well, **worry no more!** In your hands (or on your screen) is **The Quick and Easy Guide to Baby Showers.**   Within the following pages, you'll learn everything that you need to know to throw a *perfect* baby shower. You'll learn about the elements of:

> ➢ **Planning a Baby Shower from the Ground Up**

> ➢ **Managing a Baby Shower from Start to End**

> ➢ **Other Tips, Strategies, and Suggestions**

Don't worry if you've never organized a baby shower before. And worry even *less* if, in the past, you've tried to organize a baby shower but bumped into some obstacles along the way. This book is designed to be easy, practical, and fun. In fact, if you aren't careful, you may just become a baby shower *specialist*, with people calling you up and asking you for your advice and insights. Now would *that* be fun?

As you make your way through this book, bear in mind that the suggestions in here are meant to be applied – and they *do* work – but there's always an element of uniqueness to every baby shower.

So instead of putting together a baby shower in the way you might put together a recipe – adding ingredients exactly as they're listed and ending up with a predictably tasty dish – you're gently advised to approach your baby shower project a little differently. Use the advice in here as a guide for creating a magical day for the mother-to-be, and the caring people who attend the baby shower.

Some of the ideas in here you'll want to take to the bank; others might not fit with what you're trying to do, or what can be done (such as some of the baby shower games we talk about). Don't worry if you apply only some of what you read here.

Use your common sense, and remember: baby showers are supposed to be *fun* and *special* events. They aren't meant to be stressful, and the last person who should feel overwhelmed is you.

Now that you have this book, pulling together an excellent and memorable baby shower might be the easiest thing you do all year (or course, you don't have to *tell* people it was so easy...☺).

PART 1: PLANNING THE SHOWER

Who'll Throw the Shower?

There's an ongoing debate – that can actually become quite emotional and vocal – that tried to determine whether or not a relative should throw the baby shower. Traditionally, the view has been that a relative should *not* throw a baby shower, because it can appear that the relative is requesting gifts. Yet traditions change, and there are times when a sibling, or a cousin, or an aunt might be the ideal and somewhat convenient choice.

So what should you do? To answer this, we can respond with the best, and sometimes most unsatisfying answer of them all: *it depends*.

Sorry, but it really *does* depend. If you hail from a rather traditional or conventional background, it may be wise to see that a non-relative is in charge of the baby shower. In addition, even if you, personally, are comfortable with a relative throwing the baby shower, some of your guests – who may be less comfortable with it than you – may object (or just whisper about it behind your back).

Use your judgment here. Perhaps the most practical advice is this: if you can conveniently and pleasantly *not* have a relative run things, then that will likely be the best route to go. However, if that's just not possible, plausible, or preferred, then don't feel like you're someone from outer space because you're related to the mother-to-be. More and more people are breaking with tradition; especially since they feel that the perception of a relative *"asking for gifts"* arguably doesn't exist anymore.

Gifts (which we talk about further on in this book) are rather integral to baby showers; it's quite hard to imagine one *without* gifts. Since that is the case, whether a relative requests them from those attending the baby shower, or a non-relative requests them, arguably isn't important to those attending. They're likely focused on what the baby shower *should* focus on: the mother-to-be, and a wonderful opportunity to share in her joy.

Now, there's an amusing (at least from our current detached perspective) on this that you should know about. Some people may not *want* to run the baby shower. It's assumed that if you're reading this, that you're quite happy with the assignment, and you'd like to do some quality – and easy! – research so that everything goes off without a hitch.

Yet if you aren't the one whose holding the baby shower, but perhaps the mother-to-be who is about to hand over this book to a relative or friend who *will* hold the shower, then we should take a little time-out to talk about something important.

A baby shower is a wonderful event that is filled with laughter, love, and perhaps a few tears (of happiness). Yet putting one together can require an investment of time. Not *a lot* of time; not compared to, say, planning a wedding or for some people, planning a vacation.

Yet it's fair to simply note that putting together a baby shower *does* require some focus, and some time. If you're about to nominate someone to take on this task, then please bear this in mind; that person should understand that they'll need to do a little bit of work (but it's *fun* work, of course).

And if you've been asked to put together a baby shower – or if it's just been assumed that you'll do it – and you're a little worried about your own lack of time available, then *don't worry*. This book will help you immensely. Furthermore, *nothing* is stopping you from recruiting a deputy or two to help you with the details, such as preparing food, refreshments, and helping with decorations and games.

When Should the Shower Happen?

This is an important question to ask, and of course, to answer. And as usual, there are a few different viewpoints on when to hold the baby shower. Fortunately, however, these views aren't as *debatable* as they sometimes are when it comes to whether a relative or non-relative should hold the baby shower (as we discussed above). So don't worry; this is a rather easy and straightforward challenge to solve.

Now, the real problem here is simply that there *isn't* a clear answer to the question: *when should the shower happen?* The answer to this will almost always depend on factors that are specific to the mother-to-be, the guests, and other issues.

So rather than providing a "one-size-fits-all" answer here – which is something that we *can't* do without knowing the details of your particular baby shower – let's just look at the variables. Once you know these, you'll easily be able to determine when the baby shower should be held.

The Mother-to-Be

Let's start with mother-to-be. She may have a preference about when the shower should be held; and this preference should be heeded. The father-to-be might also provide input here, which is wonderful and should be part of the overall decision-making process (we take a closer look at "couples" baby-showers later on in this book).

What kinds of things might influence a mother-to-be's preference on when the shower should be held? Some of them prefer to have the shower when they're *showing*; they may feel that there's something more *appropriate* (for lack of a better word) about holding a shower when people can actually see that a baby is on the way.

In practical terms, this means that a shower might be held well into the second trimester, or into the third.

The Guests

As we all know, December is a season for parties and events; both business, and personal. As a result, it may be polite to *not* hold the baby shower during "party season", as it may influence whether people would be able to attend (or be able to *relax* when they attend, because they don't have three more "*get togethers*" to go to after the baby shower!).

Furthermore, if you live in a wintry climate, it may be a pleasant idea to *not* have the baby shower in the dead of winter. True, life does go on in the middle of January and people go to work and do many of the things that they want to do (go shopping, go to restaurants, and so on), but if it makes absolutely no difference to you and the mother-to-be (and/or the father-to-be) whether the baby shower is held in late January or late April, then it may be advisable to choose the latter; simply for climate concerns.

The Gifts

This is one that most people don't think about until someone brings it up, and then they say to themselves: *ohhhh, yes, that makes sense!* Fortunately for you, you're getting a sneak-peak at that thought well before someone at the baby shower asks it!

As we all know, some people prefer to give gender-specific gifts. While, indeed, times have changed and makers of baby-related items are creating more gender-neutral items, there's still a large contingent of people who want to give baby blue gifts to an impending son, or pink gifts to an impending daughter.

In light of this, if the parents-to-be have decided to learn the baby's gender via ultrasound, and further decided to share that information with the world-at-large, then it may be *very* appreciated by the baby shower guests if you hold the shower *after* the baby's gender information has widely disseminated. In other words: some people will be grateful that they know whether a boy or girl is on the way *before* they buy their gift.

Ultrasound gender diagnostic tests typically happen around the 9 week mark of gestation (though it can be later in some cases), and so this factor may influence whether you hold the shower early on, or wait until this information is known (assuming, of course, that the parents-to-be want to know!).

Post-Birth Baby Showers

Some people are surprised to learn that many baby showers happen *after* the baby has been born. Actually, this is quite common because, in addition to having the shower itself, this timing affords guests the wonderful opportunity to actually *see* the baby (and make all kinds of *goo goo gaa gaa* noises that we all love to make!).

Holding a post-birth shower may also work out better in light of other factors noted above, such as climate, and preferences of the parents-to-be.

Sending out Invitations

Okay, here's where things can be a little bit awkward. Scratch that; here's where some people *dread* being in charge of a baby shower, because at issue is: **who to invite?**

A good rule of thumb here is to work with the mother (and ideally, the father) to-be in order to decide who should attend, and who should be left off the list. This is a delicate scenario and can cause a number of minor headaches (even some major ones).

The problem is, simply, that while it would be ideal to invite everyone who would want to attend, that's just not practical; either economically, or simply in terms of planning. Ultimately, decisions will have to be made, and if you can work with the parents-to-be to make these decisions, the chances of making wise ones will increase.

Once you've figured out who to invite – and this process can take a few days of thinking and re-thinking – the next step is to send out the invitations. Ensure that you do this *well* in advance of the baby shower. There are two major reasons for this.

Firstly, you want to give your invitees enough lead time to that if they *do* have something planned on the baby shower date that they can, if they wish, move those plans in order to attend. If you don't provide them with enough notice, even if they *want* to change their existing plans, they might not be able to.

Secondly, you want to give people enough time to RSVP (i.e. confirm their attendance). Some people are not *the most organized people in the world*, and as such they might not RSVP right away. As such, you want to give them a bit of time to get to this on their ever-growing *TO-DO* list.

Now, there's another issue here that we should discuss. Some people think, or just assume really, that if you *don't* RSVP, that means you aren't attending. That's actually not technically correct. RSVP doesn't mean (even in the French language from where it comes) that someone is going to attend. It simply means: *please get back to me on this*.

So what's the issue? It's that it can be a little disastrous to assume that if you *don't* get an RSVP, that people won't attend. Because some people will simply show up, and when you say that you assumed they weren't coming because they didn't "RSVP", they may frown and say what we're pointing out here: RSVP, itself, doesn't mean *yes or no*. It just means: please respond.

Naturally, of course, people *should* RSVP and let you know if they're going to attend. It's the polite thing to do, without question. But *polite* is one of those *eye of the beholder* terms; and people who haven't invested several days of their life to putting a memorable baby shower together may not realize how *impolite* they are being by just showing up, unannounced.

So how do you solve this problem? Well, like all good solutions: you head it off before it *becomes* a problem! While you want to have all of your invitees RSVP, you should make it utterly clear that you'd like a response *regardless of whether they will attend*. To that end, depending on the size of your baby shower guest list, you should include a self-addressed stamped envelope and a self-typed note with each invitation that says something like this:

Dear Mary,

You are warmly invited to attend a baby shower for our friend Darla!

The shower will be held on April 15th at 1:30pm. It will be held at my home, which is at 123 Main Street. It's just one block east of Main and 8th Avenue, and ample parking is available on the street. If you need directions, please call me at 555-1234.

We'd like to have a sense of how many of Darla's friends will be able to attend. Could you please fill out this form below by checking in the appropriate box, and then mail it to me in the self-addressed stamped envelope provided? Please Send it to me by March 28th. Thank you so much!

(please check one)

☐I will be attending Jane's baby shower on April 15th at 1:30pm.

☐I regretfully will not be able to attend the baby shower.

*** Remember: Please mail before March 28th in the self-addressed stamped envelope provided. THANK YOU! ***

You can create any variation of this as you want. This is just a simple little sample that highlights the things that you should ask: whether an invitee is attending, or whether an invitee *isn't*. In other words, you don't want any grey area here; you don't want any default that says: *I didn't reply, so I'm not coming*. A little note like the one above obliges, in a polite and tasteful way, your invitee to actively let you know whether they'll show up or not.

Now, if your baby shower guest list is smaller and it's feasible to do so, you may want to skip the mailing campaign and just phone people up and ask them to attend. If you have the time and the ability to do so (e.g. the guest list is small enough for you to manage), this is the preferred method. It gives your invitees the opportunity to ask pertinent questions, such as whether the mother-to-be is in any gift registry. Let's talk about this right now.

To Gift Registry or Not to Gift Registry

This is another one of those fun decisions that involve the mother-to-be, and probably the father-to-be, as well. Gift registries are, generally speaking, *wonderful* inventions because the conveniently solve a lot of potentially confusing problems, such as:

- **What will the parents-to-be want as a gift?**

- **What gift items have already been purchased by other invitees?**

- **What price range is appropriate?**

So with all of this evidence in favor of gift registries, why might someone not use one? Well, there are few reasons.

The simplest reason is one of *preference*. Some people simply don't want to limit the range of things that guests might buy; especially if some gifts aren't typically found in stores that offer registries. For example, some artistic guests may want to *create* something for the baby; perhaps wooden mobile, or a beautiful picture to hang in the baby's room.

These kinds of items, by definition, can't appear on a gift registry; and so parents-to-be might wish to avoid using one.

Another reason is one of cost. Depending on the number of people invited to the baby shower, and presuming that those that have been invited attend, there may be a slight awkwardness if the registry contains gift possibilities that might frankly be outside of a person's price range. This can indeed be awkward.

For example, if 20% of the gifts in the registry are below, say, $30, there is some possibility that these ones will be *snatched up first*; thus leaving a latecomer to buy something more expensive, or risk buying something that isn't on the registry at all and therefore might not be wanted by the parents.

To help deal with this situation, it's possible for you (as the organizer) for informally recommend that people *band together* to buy certain bigger ticket items, like a crib or a stroller. In this way, people can still stay within their budget limitations, yet purchase something that the parents want, and indeed, need (since babies can be *very* expensive!).

Remember, of course, that if you choose the registry route, that you provide *all* the necessary details. It may also be wise to include your phone number if anyone *has any questions about gifts or the registry*.

The handful of people who may be stuck with the expensive gifts may all call you around the same time, and you can tactfully suggest that they all get together and purchase an expensive item. Voila: **problem solved!!**

PART 2: HOLDING THE SHOWER

Okay. You've figured out when to hold the shower, who to invite, and whether or not to use a gift registry. So that's all there is to it, right? *Hardly!*

Actually, you've done quite a bit of work (applaud yourself!). But there's still more work to do. Now you're really into the zone, and it's time to figure out what you're going to do *at* the shower.

Now, this may seem like a strange section. After all, people will show up at the shower, they'll hug, smile, laugh, cry (joyfully, of course), and have a good time. That part is taken care of. Yet there's more to it than this.

In addition to the natural events that are going to occur at the baby shower, you want to continue managing *during* the shower. In other words, you want to have things for your invitees to do, and for them to drink/eat.

Let's look at each of these important aspects below.

Things to Do: Themes

In case you haven't been a baby shower lately, here's some useful information for you: **themes are in**!

This means that more and more people are opting to create a certain style, or *theme*, of baby shower. Do you remember those high school dances that were built around a theme? Like oldies theme, or rock & roll theme, or something else? And the decorations and so forth all reflected the chosen theme? Well, that's the same deal here with thematic baby showers.

Now, the sky truly is the limit on what theme you'd like to use. Really: anything that you can imagine, provided that it's realistic and within your budget, is fine.

To create a theme, simply have the following items reflect what you've chosen:

☑ **the invitations should themselves reflect the chosen theme (e.g. Alice in Wonderland)**

☑ **the baby shower room should be decorated with items reflecting the theme (e.g. colors, posters, props such as stuffed animals or balloons)**

☑ **the refreshments and food (discussed further in this book) should reflect the theme.**

Now, just in case you want to get your creative juices flowing, some suggested themes are provided to you below. They're all from the website www.babycenter.com, and from *real people* who held successful baby showers (just like yours will be!).

Theme: A Tea Party

Do you remember playing *tea party* when you were a child? You'd get together with your little friends, or perhaps your stuffed animals (who were alive, of course), and together you sat down and enjoyed a pleasant and lighthearted chat over a cup of tea.

Back then, it's possible that your tea was, well, of the *invisible* variety. After all, you weren't allowed to have boiling water in your pot; you might burn yourself! Now, however, you're all grown up and can enjoy the *visible* variety of tea (it tastes a little different).

To enjoy this theme, simply re-create that vision of when you were young. Invite all of your stuffed animals (who are *still* alive, of course), and have them sit in chairs around the area where the baby shower is being held (probably the living room or perhaps a finished basement).

This theme is sure to bring back a lot of warm memories for all of your guests; because most of us did play *at tea* a few times. To that end, you can invite each guest to bring a stuffed animal who can attend the festivities (and they can even leave the stuffed animal behind as a little bonus gift for the baby!).

Theme: Celebrity

Really: who wouldn't like feeling like a celebrity every now and then? Imagine, having people around you bustling to get your autograph, or to take a picture of you for those glamour magazines...ah, what a life.
The celebrity here, however, isn't going to be you (sorry), or even the mother-to-be. It's going to be her baby! So this theme calls for decorations that are worthy of a star – perhaps even a big Hollywood sign out on the lawn, or in the front hallway.

And the invitations, too, can be publicity releases instead of traditional invitations, announcing the coming out of Hollywood's next rising star.

And, of course, don't forget the cake! Instead of a regular cake, you can have one shaped like a star – like on the Hollywood Walk of Fame! All of these little elements help add humor and energy to the baby shower, and further ensure that it's a memorable experience for everyone, especially the mother-to-be.

Theme: Literary Baby

It doesn't matter what kind of childhood we had, or how often we found ourselves curled up reading that very first book that made such a positive impression on our growing imaginations. It could have been a *Dr. Seuss* book, or perhaps something a bit later, such as your first *Nancy Drew Mystery*.

Regardless, a literary theme baby shower calls for each guest to bring (in addition to their gift) a *special book* from their childhood; something that inspired them and, indeed, continues to hold a fond place in their heart after all of these years.

Though it'll be a number of years before the baby learns to read any of the books, they will serve as a wonderful library that the child can grow into; especially since each book has been chosen with such great care and affection.

Of additional value, having a literary theme is a *fantastic* ice breaker. It gives everyone a chance to share *why* the book was so special to them.

Chances are, there will be a lot of nodding, and smiling, and maybe even a few tears, too (the good kind, of course!).

Things to Do: Games

Baby showers are *ideal* places to play games. They not only help break the ice and get people laughing, but since baby showers are about having fun: what's more fun than a good game? It's better than working, right!

There are several games that you can play, ranging from old standards like charades, to more modern ideas like trivia games. A trip to your local toy store will fill you with several ideas of what could work.

However, you may feel like creating a game that has a kind of special *baby shower feel* to it; something that is entertaining and mildly competitive, but ties into the fact that it's being played at a baby shower.

So in light of that, here are some great baby shower-specific games that come to us from geniusbabies.com (http://www.geniusbabies.com/babshowgam1.html). You can alter these games in any way that you wish to specifically suit your theme.

Game: The Winning Plate

This neat little game involves what most people love in life: **food!** Simply put a picture of a baby beneath one of the plates that will be handed out to guests as they eat.   Don't tell anyone that the picture is there; just let them eat. When the eating part of the event is coming to a close, tell your guests to peek under their plate, and give the lucky guest who has the picture a prize!

Game: The Price is Right

People seem to *love* this game, because it's based on what many feel is the best game show of all time: The Price is Right!

Simply purchase a number of baby items, such as diapers, baby food, a pacifier, or anything that can be found in an ordinary neighborhood grocery store. Then, have the guests *bid* on how much they think everything cost. Reward each winning bidder with a prize; or offer them points, and then total up the points at the end. The winner of the overall game can then win a prize.

Game: That... Was ME?

This is a tremendously enjoyable game! Invite each guest to bring a baby picture of *themselves*. Collect each picture, and then put them on a giant board. During the baby shower, allow guests to go up and browse the big board of pictures.

Provide each guest with a piece of paper and a pen/pencil, and have them write down the names of who they think each picture is (put a number beside each picture so that they can be referenced).

At the end of the game, reveal the answers and see who has the best eye! This game is not only slightly competitive, but it also always leads to a lot of laughs and *ohhhh you were so cuuuuuuute*'s!

Food

Author Randy Wilson (http://ezinearticles.com/?Baby-Shower-Food-Items&id=42045) has put together a wonderful article on the importance of food at the baby shower. He also delivers some fantastic advice on what to choose; and what *not* to choose.

The first thing that Wilson wisely notes is that a full course meal really isn't typical for a baby shower. Rather, finger-foods, appetizers, and munchies like chips and crackers are more common. A cake is also rather common, as are other deserts, such as ice creams and pies. If you're going to splurge on any of the items, then going a bit extra on the deserts is usually considered the more acceptable approach. After all, who doesn't love cake?

Also, as noted above, the foods in the baby shower can tie into the theme. If the theme is *celebrity*, for example, then the sandwiches can be in the shape of little stars. The foods don't *have* to reflect the theme; which means that you should feel bad, or like a failure, if you can't find a way to make little star-shaped sandwiches (it really is an art form!). However, if you can tie everything together, it will make your baby shower that much more memorable an event for the guests, and the parents-to-be.

Having a wide selection is also important; and we discuss this in some detail in the "Insider's Tips" section of this book. Suffice it to say, try and have enough variety to account for tastes *and* dietary preferences. Nowadays, the wise approach is often to allow guests to do a little bit of preparing themselves.

For example, instead of putting the salad dressing in the salad, or putting condiments such as mayonnaise on the finger sandwiches, you can leave these for your guests to add themselves, if they so choose.

The same goes for deserts. While it's wonderful to have rich cake and tasty pies available, it's always nice to offer fruit as an alternative. Some people may not want to (or may not be allowed to!) consume that many calories, or enjoy that much sugar.

PART 3: INSIDER'S TIPS

Ah yes. What would a how-to book be without insider's tips? These are the tried, tested, and sometimes *regrettable* details that you really **need to know** in order to create, management, and complete a perfect baby shower.

You'll likely find some of these to be common-sense; though a few may surprise you. It's these strange ones that are the most important to you, because heeding the advice – to do or *not* to do them – can be the difference between making your baby shower memorable for the right reasons, or for the wrong ones. These are all from the great website www.mamabebe.com.

As you plan and roll-out more baby showers (because you'll be so good at this one people will want to consult your services!), your list of *dos and dont's* will increase. Keep a journal handy to jot these insights and experienced down as you go.

Things to Do: Plan

It goes without saying (but let's say it anyway, since we're all here together!). PLEASE PLAN AHEAD!

You may be one of those very talented people who tend to do things without a lot of planning; you just have a *flair* for pulling things off, and often, for pulling them *out* just in the nick of time. If this sounds like you, then you should really heed these sage word: **PLEASE PLAN AHEAD**!

The thing about a baby shower is that there are a lot of variables that come together to determine whether it succeeds or doesn't succeed. As you know from reading the first section in this book, everything from choosing the time of year for the shower, to the amount of time to "RSVP" the invitations, are elements that *can influence* the shower. Or to put things more frankly: if something is *wrong* in any of these elements, then they will almost certainly negatively influence the overall baby shower experience.

So how do you deal with this? Simply by *planning ahead*.
Have a plan – write it out! – and see what you have to do,
and in what timeframe. If you need help, then talk to the
mother-to-be and recruit some deputies. If you need
assistance making a decision – such as who to invite – then
get the help that you need. By *planning*, you're able to see
what you need to do, and therefore, you can go ahead and
do it.

On the flipside, when you *don't* plan, you are almost
certainly going to overlook a detail or two. At the time, they
may seem minor ("do I *really* need to follow-up with people
who haven't RSVP'd the invitation?").

Yet once the shower actually happens, it's kind of like racing
a car in the Indy 500: if there are flaws, they will be
exposed. So don't let your little details come back to bite
you, or any of the other guests (including the mother-to-
be).

If you aren't a good planner, then here's your opportunity to
become one. It's not that hard at all; it just requires a little
effort (that goes a long way!).

Things to Do: Decorate

One of the most *memorable* things about the baby shower will be the decorations. They might seem like yet another minor detail in a sea of details, but they will be something that people notice, appreciate, and indeed, remember.

You don't have to go overboard on the decorations, and you *don't* have to spend a lot of money. In fact, the biggest investment here will probably be your time. Simply choose the decorations that reflect the theme that you've chosen. You may want to consult the mother-to-be on the decorations.

For example, if the mother-to-be is deathly afraid of spiders, a *Charlotte's Web* theme with giant spider decorations probably isn't the wisest decision to make.

Things to Do: Cater Accordingly

Perhaps more than ever before, people are very serious about what they eat; and what they don't. In the past, it was somewhat safe to make catering decisions based on religious or cultural understanding.

For instance, many Catholics don't eat red meat on Friday. As such, if the guest list included people who you knew followed this practice, you would simply include non red-meat alternatives, such as seafood. Or if your guests were Jewish, you wouldn't serve pork.

While these cultural catering rules still certainly apply, more people these days are choosing to eat based on lifestyle choices, not just religious or spiritual ones. Many people, for example, don't eat foods that contain trans-fats. Or many people don't eat foods that are high in carbohydrates, or proteins (it's hard to tell which one is good these days, and which one is bad!). There are also many more practicing vegetarians in the western world right now; and that, too, can be a little confusing. Some people who describe themselves as vegetarians will eat fish. Some will drink milk. Some won't eat cheese or honey.

For fun, log onto the website of any international airline, like American Airways or Delta, for example. And within their site, just check out the *in-flight hospitality* section to see the different kinds of meals that are available. You'll be

amazed at how many different categories of food there are. You'll find everything from low-calorie to lacto-vegetarian, to low-carbohydrate to low-sodium, and even more.

Now, don't worry: you don't have to serve *dozens* of kinds of food! The idea here is simply to be aware that in the world today, people are much more informed about what they'll eat; and what they won't.

So when you make your catering decisions, try and *think outside of the box* a little. This means, see if any choices that you're making could limit your guests' enjoyment of a particular food. For example, if you're ordering little finger sandwiches, it may be wise to have cold cuts on a separate plate that people can pick and choose from at their discretion. Those who don't want cold cuts (for any reason, including taste preference) can simply not pick them up.

Also consider the *types* of foods that you offer. If your guest list is going to be predominantly filled with senior citizens, foods like celery – which are murder on dentures! – isn't a good idea.

Before we go onto the next *do*, please take a moment to consider whether you'll have alcohol at the baby shower. Now, this book is not a legal guide and nothing within it, naturally, should be seen as legal advice. However, according to media reports, there have been some cases where people at parties consumed too much alcohol and, as a result, injured themselves and other people. This is tragic enough, but to add even more unhappiness, the party hosts were also seen as partly liable.

Now, these isolated cases which have garnered so much media attention were for holiday and new year's eve-type parties, where alcohol is considered a party staple. It's hard to imagine a baby shower where anyone would drink past the point of sensible. Yet it *can* happen, and it's something that you simply need to be mindful of. So if you are going to serve alcohol of any kind – be it punch or wine or wine coolers, etc. – then make sure that you do what you *need to do* to cut people off who may not know when to stop.

Or, like many people, you can just choose to have an alcohol-free baby shower and not give it a second thought! The choice is yours (and presumably the parents-to-be), but it's something worth discussion *beforehand*.

Things to Do: Set a Time Limit

Baby showers are wonderful events filled with relaxing laughter and shared positive emotions. Yet all good things come to and end. Or rather, all good things *should* come to an end while they're still good things.

This means, simply, that you should have a clear end-time for the baby shower. This allows guests to efficiently plan their day, and it also gives everyone a chance to leave at the same time and not appear impolite for *"having to run and miss all of the fun"*.

You don't have to monitor the baby shower so that is stays precisely on schedule; this isn't a job, remember, and there are no shareholders!

While you'll certainly want to usher the baby shower through its various phases (such as moving from games to food with enough time for people to eat), the important thing here is that the baby shower should end on time.

Things NEVER to Do: Don't Choose Awkward Games

We've come a long way from *charades*. Now, there are shelves full of games specifically designed for adults. Some of these games, as you can imagine – or might have even enjoyed yourself a time or two – are of the... er...well, they can be a bit *racy*. And they can ask awkward questions and inspire awkward moments; because that's part of the fun of the game.

Now, you simply *don't* want the word "awkward" to be anywhere near your baby shower. In fact, you want to keep awkward at least 500 feet away from your baby shower at all times. So to help do this, ensure that the games you choose are suitable for everyone and won't lead to awkward situations.

Also, think even further than whether the game itself is intended for "adults only". Some games, like *Twister*, aren't typically enjoyed by people who may be obese, or who are afflicted with a physical limitation.

For example, if one of your guests is confined to a wheelchair, then having a game that requires mobility – like Twister, or a rousing rendition of *musical chairs* – can be very awkward. It can actually inspire hurt feelings.

Naturally, you can't be expected to plan ahead for every eventuality. You won't know, for instance, that one of the guests had a very traumatic *piñata* experience as a child, and therefore runs out of the room screaming when she sees one of them flying through the air. So what should you do when you can't know everything that there is to know?

Simple: just have a few options. Keep a few back-up games handy, just in case you detect that people are uncomfortable with the choices. It sounds like a little thing, but it can truly make the difference between keeping *awkward* at bay, or having it crash the baby shower.

Things NEVER to Do: Don't Ask People to Eat Standing Up

Some people like eating while standing up; particularly kids, who always seem to be on the go and ready to do the next thing. Some of them even eat *while* doing something else, like walking or talking on the phone.

However, it's safe to assume that your baby shower guests aren't going to be that *frenetic* with their movements. They'll likely want to peacefully sit down and eat; and that's why you must ensure that they have somewhere to sit, and a place to eat.

This is an oversight that a lot of very well-intentioned baby shower producers make. The thing is, it's sometimes very hard to envision just how much table and chair space is necessary. A room may look very spacious, but fill it with 15 people or more, and it can become very cramped.

Again, the solution to this is in the word *plan*. Take a good look at the space in which the baby shower will take place. Literally count the number of sitting spaces, and the number of table spaces. If there aren't enough of *both* to comfortably serve the number of people attending, then you need to do something about this.

A quick and easy solution could be renting fold-away tables and chairs that can be brought out and then put away when the food is finished. Or, if the weather is nice, you can *maybe* count on doing things outside. If you do this, however, keep in mind that some people may still want to eat inside. Furthermore, always bear in mind that weather predictions are simply that: predictions. Don't overestimate that accuracy of a sunny forecast; we've all woken up to thunderstorms on the day of the big picnic.

Also keep in mind that in western culture (e.g. American, Canadian, and some parts of Western Europe), personal space is generally seen as *larger* than those in other countries.

You can visibly see this if you ride the subway in, say, New York compared to Tokyo. When possible, the New Yorkers will allow for about 2 feet of personal space around each person. Of course, in rush hour this isn't possible, but otherwise the 2-foot-rule is generally held.

In Tokyo, however, the personal space expectations are around 1 foot; regardless of density of the subway car. People in Japan are simply more comfortable with a 1 foot personal space orbit, while people in the US are simply more comfortable with a 2+ foot orbit.

What does this mean to you?   It means that you should be *aware* of the personal space needs of your guests; because if you aren't, then they'll be uncomfortable. So even if you believe you have enough room to seat and feed 15 people, ask yourself: is this *really* the case? Or are you literally cramming people to sit and eat side by side in a manner that is going to be culturally uncomfortable?

It's little things like this that may seem like superficial details, but in fact, they make a *huge* difference when the baby shower actually happens. So if you don't really have enough space, then take steps to find more space; or, at the very least, don't serve foods like soups that require a stable eating area (firm chair and firm table).

If you absolutely can't find enough space for all of the guests, choose foods like dry sandwiches that people can eat as they stand, or sit on a stairwell.

Obviously, the ideal is to have *everyone* sit. But if you can't, then your choice of catering can make things as good as they can be, all things considered.

Couples Showers?

The website www.preggiepeggy.com has an amusing article on what many call *co-ed baby showers*. This term doesn't actually mean that couples should be invited to baby showers. Rather, it refers to the *husband* of the mother-to-be inviting *his* friends to the baby shower.

A very good trend over the last generation or so is that more men are participating in the whole childbirth experience. Many men are now also involved in the birth itself, assisting the mother with coaching and helping her endure the stress. In this light, it's not strange to imagine that men are participating in baby showers in unprecedented numbers.

The decision to have men at the baby shower – and these would be friends of the father – is a decision that, naturally, would be made by both would-be parents. It's nothing that the baby shower producer (you!) should assume; because there may be pros and cons about the wisdom of this co-ed option.

If you decide to invite men, then *ensure* that this is reflected on the invitation. Also, keep in mind that many men consider Sunday to be a *holy day* in more than just religious terms. During football season (October through to January), Sunday is a very important day for *many* men; and showing up to a shower might be the last thing that they want to do.

So just bear this in mind, and if you *have* to do things on a Sunday, make sure that it isn't Super Bowl Sunday! And there's a period in March affectionately called *March Madness*; it's a very special time for many men (and women!).

If you're not sure of when these special moments are, consult with your local sports nut. They'll be able to tell you when high and low season are!

Also keep in mind that some of the feminine elements of a traditional baby shower – such as, perhaps, the Tea Party theme – should probably go out the window if you're doing things co-ed. Find something entertaining and, if at all possible, gender neutral.

Remember too that, just due to cultural upbringing, many men aren't into the *dainty* side of life. So while they'll gladly attend to support their friend (the father-to-be), don't expect them to get all teary eyed as they discuss why *Little Women* was the most important book in their life.

CONCLUSION

Take a breath, and give yourself a round of applause. You now know more about planning the *perfect* baby shower than most people ever will.

For instance, you now know the importance of planning everything from the timing of the shower, to the food being served, to whether there's enough space for people to eat and sit comfortably.

You also know about *themes* and *games* that can make the baby shower a memorable and joyous event for all. And, of course, you know about some of the essential *do's* and *dont's* that can make all of the difference in determining whether a baby shower succeeds, or runs into some trouble along the way.

Remember, as we pointed out at the very beginning of this book, your vision here in planning the perfect baby shower should be a flexible vision; there is no guaranteed prescription that will magically lead to the perfect experience.

Each baby shower has its own unique aspects, and there's really on way to predict what will happen.

However, by following the proven, simple, and clear advice in this book, you'll put yourself *way* ahead of the pack and truly hit the ground running.

- ➢ While others fail to understand why playing *Taboo* was an error, the guests at the baby shower that you put together will not have that problem.

- ➢ While others try and force their guests to eat hot soup without a table to rest it on, your guests will enjoy sandwiches that *travel nicely*.

- ➢ While other bore their guests, your guests will be laughing and having a good time thanks to the themes and games that you've provided.

➢ While others put together a baby shower that lacks character and uniqueness, people will rave about the one you put together for years to come.

➢ While others commit the cardinal sin of inviting men to a baby shower on Super Bowl Sunday, or during the Sweet 16 of the NCAA Basketball tournament when the local university is playing, you'll have people sending you thank you cards for your *consideration* in scheduling things around that important day.

...and the list goes on, and on, and on!

Good luck, have fun, and remember: baby showers are about sharing good times and having fun! Keep this in mind, and there is no problem or challenge that you can't overcome.

And don't forget to keep a journal of your experiences – both positive and not-so-positive. This can serve both as a priceless *memento* of your baby shower experience, and as a very useful tool for you as you go to your next baby shower; or help someone plan *their* perfect event!

www.ingramcontent.com/pod-product-compliance
Lightning Source LLC
Chambersburg PA
CBHW050834290526
45792CB00001B/387